THE **ARM** BOOK

ARM PAIN

- keep active to recover quickly
- this booklet tells you how

London: TSO

First published 2011

Single copy ISBN 9780117069145

Pack of 10 copies (ISBN 9780117069138)

Discounts apply for larger quantities. Call 0870 600 5522

Also available from TSO

- 'The Back Book' (ISBN 9780117029491) offering advice to those with lower back pain.
- 'Get Back Active' (ISBN 9780117039360) a DVD based on the Back Book giving practical guidance on handling back pain
- 'The Whiplash Book' (ISBN 9780117028623) offering advice on how to deal with a whiplash injury - based on the latest research
- 'The Neck Book' (ISBN 9780117033214) offering advice to those affected by neck pain
- 'Your Back Operation' (ISBN 9780117038332) helping people recover from a back operation.
- 'Health & Work' (9780117037625) advising people with common health problems to stay at work or get back quickly.

Illustrations by Rachel Oxley

Printed in the United Kingdom for The Stationery Office

WHY THE ARM BOOK?

So you've got pain in your arm – it may be anywhere from the shoulder to the fingertips. You're not alone. In fact most people get pain in their upper limbs at some stage during their lives.

Like most others you're probably uncertain about whether to rest, whether to seek treatment, and whether to go to work. Probably you're also worried about what's going on and what the future holds.

The Arm Book is here to answer these and other questions in terms you can understand – no jargon, just sound information and advice. It tells you what you need to know to get back to what you usually do. It also tells you what to expect, from whom, and when.

WHO IS IT FOR?

This booklet is for people with painful arm problems. The sort of conditions you'll have heard about such as tennis elbow, carpal tunnel syndrome, or frozen shoulder. Actually, they have a lot of similarities, and are often bundled together under the term upper limb disorders.

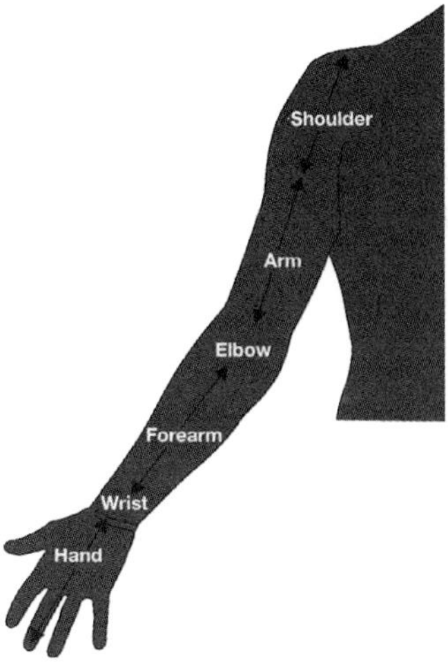

The focus of the following advice is about helping you manage things and getting on with life. How you do this is pretty much always the same, no matter why you got arm pain in the first place.

You may need treatment, or you may not. Most pain gets better on its own, but some types of arm pain certainly do need treatment from a doctor or therapist.

The trick is to make best use of that treatment so you can stay active. It really is important you understand this, so you don't fall into the trap of avoiding all activity.

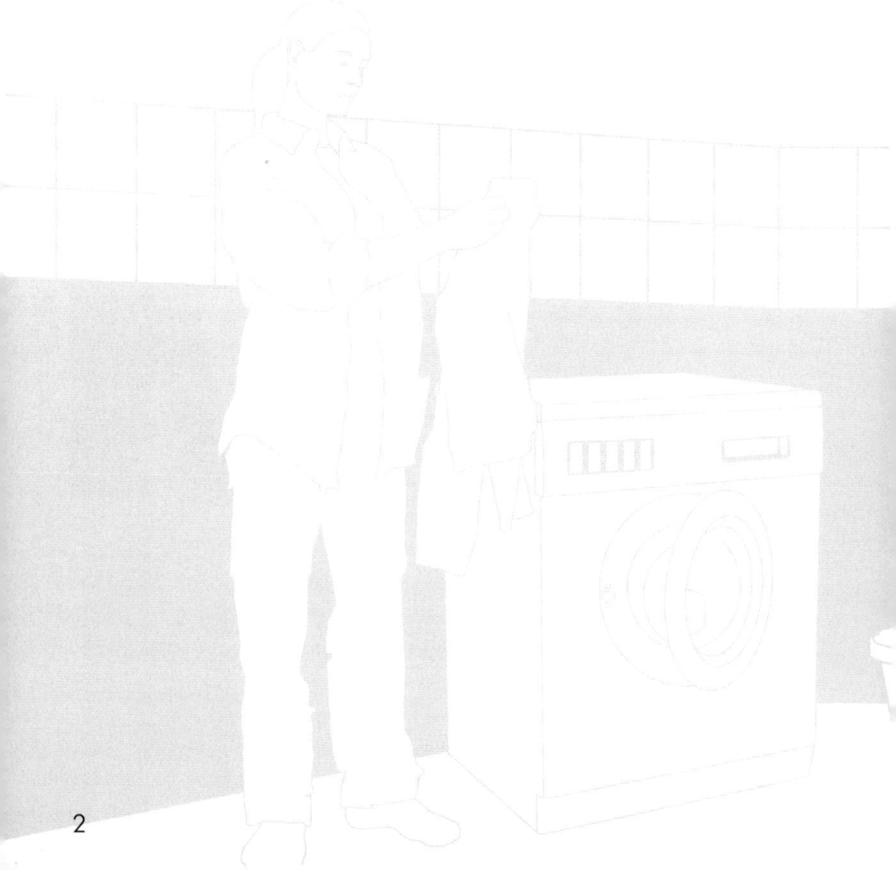

CAUSES AND EFFECTS

So, what might have happened to cause your pain? You're bound to be curious, but most times you'll find you get different explanations from different people! So far as getting on with things is concerned, it actually doesn't matter too much what's gone wrong.

Arm pain can be triggered, or set off, by all sorts of everyday activities. People sometimes recall a specific incident like a wrench or a bump, but often there is no obvious single event or activity. In many cases it's most likely to be a combination of things.

The chances are that the pain is coming from soft-tissues around the joints – muscles, ligaments, tendons. Think of it like a strain or sprain.

That means parts of the arm may be sore to the touch or may be very painful to move for a while. The muscles may hurt when you use them, and things may stiffen up.

You may find you simply cannot do certain things for a while, such as reaching up because your shoulder is stiff or lifting the kettle because your elbow is painful. However, there are lots of other things you will be able to do just fine, so carry on doing them – being active won't be harmful.

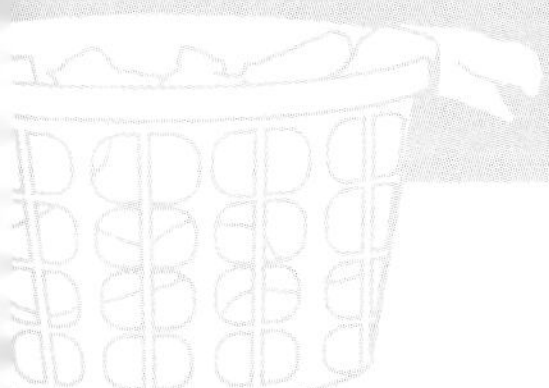

Sometimes pain is more severe than it is at other times. It may seem to spread and appear in different parts of the arm. Because that's the way our nervous system works, it isn't anything to worry about. It's really not unusual to have a lot of pain without any permanent damage.

Labels

There are dozens of commonly used labels for arm pain. Most of them relate to a medical diagnosis, but doctors don't always agree on these labels or on what causes the problems, especially in the early stages. This means the label you're given may be quite general - for instance, the term tennis elbow tends to be used as a generic label for various elbow problems.

Other labels are not medical and are frankly unhelpful. The classic example is so-called 'RSI' (repetitive strain injury). Science has shown that people with arm pain that is put down to 'RSI' do not have a strain or an injury, and often have not done anything repetitive! The term 'RSI' is misleading in that it suggests you should avoid movement and activity. As you read this booklet you'll see that inactivity is not the best way forward.

The individual conditions affecting the arms can be rather difficult to disentangle. For our purposes they can be grouped around each of the joints, because the way you can best deal with them is much the same. Here are a few examples you may come across:

Shoulder: frozen shoulder; impingement syndrome; rotator cuff injury; tendonitis......

Elbow: tennis elbow, golfer's elbow, epicondylitis......

Wrist and hand: de Quervains; tenosynovitis; carpal tunnel syndrome; triger finger; ganglion......

The diagnosis – the medical term for your condition – may be important to your doctor or therapist of course. They need to understand the problem in order to work out whether you need specific treatment to relieve your symptoms. It is important to understand that you have a soft-tissue problem, not a serious injury. There are many causes for these problems. The way to speed your recovery and get back to your usual activities is pretty much the same whatever the diagnosis.

Arm pain is often given a label:
Tennis elbow; teno, RSI etc.

The label doesn't matter that much – it's what you do about it that counts:

... and that means doing things as normally as possible

... and that applies whatever label you've been given!

Work and arm pain

Arm pain is often not caused by work. Yet work can be difficult or painful because of it. We'll advise you what to do about this a bit later on.

You've probably heard that repetitive or strenuous work causes arm pain, or that arm pain at work is due to a build up of strain over months or years. We now know that this is not what usually happens. Most people do the same job for years without any problem.

This is important because if you mistakenly believe the activities you do at work are the cause of your arm pain then you'll be tempted to stay away from work. And that won't be helpful.

There are a couple of conditions linked to specific types of job. Yet they can also result from everyday situations, and are sometimes associated with normal aging.

Tenosynovitis: is thought to be an inflammation of the tendons of the forearm or hand. It's sometimes seen in people whose work involves frequent or repeated movements of the hand or wrist. However, most people doing that sort of work do **not** get tenosynovitis.

Carpal tunnel syndrome: is due to compression of the nerves at the front of the wrist. It is thought to occur in some people whose work involves using vibrating hand-held power tools or repeatedly bending the wrist up and down. However, most people who do that sort of work do **not** get carpal tunnel syndrome.

Remember, in most cases, work is no more likely to be the cause of arm pain than some leisure activities. Even when your problem has been triggered by a work activity, which happens sometimes, it is unlikely to result in serious injury. It would be a mistake to think the work must have been dangerous just because you experienced or developed pain while at work. We'll talk about working safely with arm pain later on.

FACTS ABOUT ARM PAIN

Now seems a good time to summarise the main facts about arm pain.

- Arm pain is a frequent experience -
  - it is generally short-lived but can happen again
  - it is often triggered by a physical strain (minor over-exertion):
    - due to everyday activities, including work
    - it hardly ever involves serious damage
  - some cases need treatment, but many settle with self-management:
    - activity is usually helpful: prolonged rest is not
  - you can expect recovery and early return to your usual activities and work:
    - lasting effects are uncommon
- There is a lot you can do to help yourself -
  - many people don't need treatment from a doctor or therapist
    - medication from the pharmacist can help

- Work is not the major cause -
  - some work can be difficult or impossible initially:
    - yet that does not mean the work is unsafe
    - blaming work is often wrong and unhelpful
  - most people manage to stay at work:
    - you may need to reduce hours or have some time off if your job mainly involves strenuous use of your arms
- Early return to work is important -
  - it contributes to the recovery process and will usually do no harm
    - getting back to work quickly requires support from both the workplace and the doctor

There are two other very important facts for you to know:

- There is little chance that the pain or discomfort can simply be 'switched off' by taking medications or having treatments. It is likely to improve gradually
- Resting and avoiding using your arm for more than a few days is generally a bad idea. Because it results in loss of flexibility and muscle strength, rest tends to do more harm than good. Of course you may need to make some changes to the way you go about doing things for a while

> - Arm pain is very common – pretty much everyone gets it from time to time
> - Most episodes settle quite quickly
> - Often there is no obvious cause or serious injury
> - Worrying about what's happened is unhelpful
> - Hurt does not mean damage or harm
> - You can do a lot to help yourself
> - Staying active is far better than resting up too much

MYTHS

There are lots of myths about soft-tissue pain: what it is, and how to deal with it. Scientific research shows that many of the stories you are likely to hear are wrong. The myths need busting. Read this booklet carefully to get the facts about your problem, and what has been proven to help.

Myth: Pain means serious damage and injury

- This is not always the case: pain can occur without injury
- Even when specific tissues are affected, activity and work are not usually taboo
- Temporary discomfort is often part of recovery

Myth: I must rest until the pain goes

- Quite the contrary – activity leads to faster and more sustained recovery and return to work
- Temporary reduction of activity may be required, but long-term rest is a bad idea

Myth: It's an injury or a health problem so there must be a cure

- Not really - most people, do not seek or need treatment for most episodes of arm problems
- Sometimes treatment is needed of course, but reliance on treatment alone is not enough to help with return to work

Myth: It hurts at work so I was damaged by work

- Arm pain is common across the whole population, regardless of type of work
- Work or activity can trigger symptoms, but most work is unlikely to cause serious damage

Myth: Working whilst I'm 'injured' is bound to make matters worse

- The actual condition is usually not made worse by continuing to work (assuming control of significant risks)
- Work can be difficult or uncomfortable, but that doesn't mean it is doing damage or making matters worse

Myth: I need time off work

- Often sick leave is not needed – staying at work is generally good – maybe you'll need some temporary help to do your job
- Ask your doc for a 'fit note' at the outset so you don't lose time off work!

Myth: Obviously I can't go back to work until 100% fixed

- Most people can, and do, get back to work with ongoing symptoms – with the right support they come to no harm

It's all too easy for the myths to take over. With what you've learned so far you'll be able to spot where things went wrong for Sam:

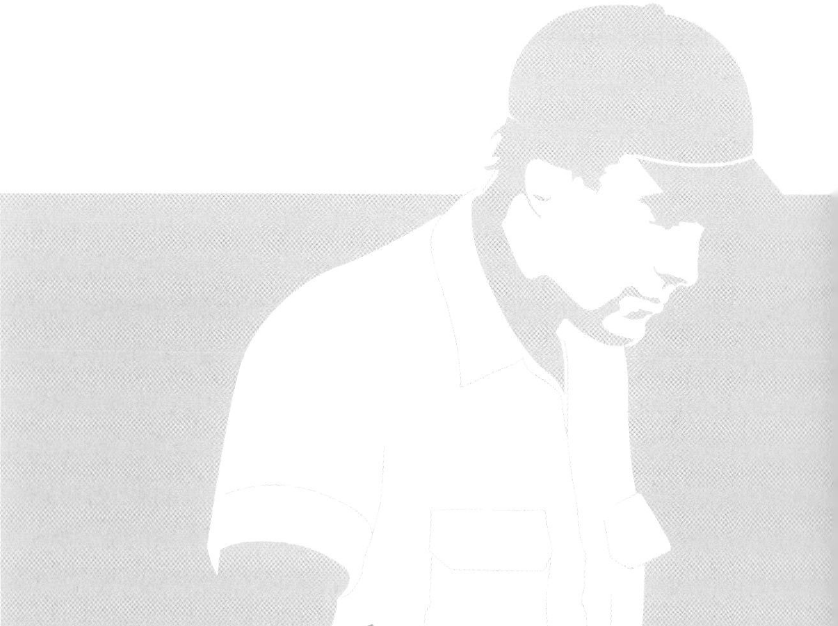

I got up one morning and had a really sore elbow. It sort of had a burning feeling so I went to see the doc and was told to take some tablets and to rest and stay off work. It didn't get any better so I was sent for x-rays, which they said showed some 'degeneration'. That was a bit scary to hear. Of course I had to wait to get treatment. When I did get to see a therapist I was told it was my job that started it, so I shouldn't go back till I was fully fixed. They couldn't tell me how long that would be so I got worried and confused. After a while I felt down in the dumps too. The family won't let me do anything; they're scared I'll get worse. I don't get out much, so I'm lonely. The people at work haven't been in touch, so I don't know what's happening about me going back. Some other people are saying I should make a claim. It's all turned into a bit of a nightmare. All I wanted was a bit of help, but now it's taken over my life...

OBSTACLES TO RECOVERY

Various things can get in the way of your recovery and can stop you getting back to work and activity. You need to spot these and do something about them if you're going to help yourself get back to your normal life. It's often helpful to talk with others about how to deal with these obstacles.

Personal obstacles involve how you feel and think:

- Unhelpful attitudes and beliefs about health and work
- Uncertainty
- Anxiety and depression
- Loss of routine and work habits

Work-related obstacles can block your return to work:

- Loss of contact with work
- Negative attitudes by people at work
- Modified work not available
- Misunderstandings and disagreements between you, your employer, and doctor/therapist

Health-related obstacles can confuse and delay:

- Conflicting advice
- Waiting lists
- Prolonged sick leave
- Ineffective treatments

Warning signs to watch out for

You'll struggle to recover and return to work if you:

- convince yourself there is something seriously wrong
- are unable to accept reassurance and help
- avoid activity in case it makes things worse
- get withdrawn and depressed
- are fearful and uncertain about going back to work

You need to make a plan to get active and working.

The key is communication and action. There are two main issues:

Recovery depends on working with the health professionals who are helping you, and on your own motivation and effort.

Treatment can help to reduce your symptoms, but you are the one who has to get active – see activity as part of the treatment.

Ask yourself: What can I do to be a 'coper' and not an 'avoider'?

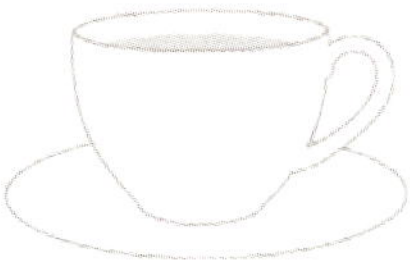

Returning to work depends on you and your employer working together, and that needs communication.

The key thing is to stay in touch with the people at work – figure out what's needed to help you return.

Ask yourself: What obstacles are getting in the way of my going back to work, and who do I need to talk to about overcoming these (by problem-solving and negotiation).

Overcoming obstacles:

- Accept reassurance and help instead of thinking there is something seriously wrong
- Focus on what you can do
- Be active, knowing that activity aids recovery

MANAGING YOUR ARM PAIN

There are three things you need to do:

- Understand your problem
- Get help to relieve symptoms
- Keep up your usual activities (including work)

Understand your problem

The first thing you need to understand is that you do **not** have a serious disease or injury. Your GP or physiotherapist can usually tell very quickly that you do not have a major problem. But, in the early stages it is difficult for them to work out exactly what's wrong. That explains some of the confusion over labels or diagnoses. Fortunately it doesn't matter too much for overall management of the vast majority of arm problems.

> **UNDERSTANDING**
>
> "The pain was so sharp when it started it felt agonising, and I thought straight away to myself this must be serious.
> I was so relieved when it soon got better – I should have realised I'd only strained things."

Once you have been reassured that you do not have a serious problem you are likely to be given a diagnosis by the doctor or physiotherapist. This will be offered as an explanation of your symptoms. Don't be frightened by the words! It's common to get different explanations and labels when you see different practitioners. This can feel confusing, and it is probably best not to focus too much on the diagnosis.

The most important thing is for you to understand that you have soft-tissue pain or discomfort, not a serious problem; and that there are many causes for these problems. However, what you do to help yourself is usually the most important factor in your recovery. This involves symptom relief, and being active.

Relieve your symptoms

You may have a variety of symptoms. The most common is pain or discomfort. However, some people get feelings such as muscle cramping, stiffness, numbness, burning, tingling, pins-and-needles, or muscle weakness.

Reducing your symptoms makes it easier to get active and will help you get on with doing the normal things in life.

For soft tissue problems the two main forms of medicine are:

RELIEVING SYMPTOMS

"I used to think that there was a cure for everything. Now I realise that my body can do a lot of its own recovery. The thing I can do to help it is being positive and applying a bit of common sense and getting some pain relief to let me do things."

- Anti-inflammatory medication (such as ibuprofen or diclofenac). This can be bought over-the-counter from the pharmacy as pills or as a gel to rub on. Both can be effective for reducing symptoms of pain and discomfort, but if your arm pain is quite localized, the gel rubbed into the painful area can be very useful
- Pain relief. You can get several types from your chemist. It is usually better to take them regularly 'by-the-clock' while you recover, and not to wait until pain builds up and is harder to control

There is no point continuing to take any medication if it does not help.

Another approach to easing the pain is to use movement to get relief: exercise and activity are good at releasing the body's natural chemicals that dull pain. You may also get relief from gentle muscle stretches or massage (another person may do this to you, or you may do it to yourself). Some people find hot or cold packs helpful.

Find what works best for you – it may be a combination of these things. Remember, controlling the pain is only part of the story. You need to combine it with activity if you are to get better quickly.

Sometimes, of course, people need additional help. If it's very painful and things are not improving in a few days, you may need some treatment.

Therapists use massage and exercises to help reduce the pain and get you going again. If you get some relief, it may be repeated a number of times while you recover. If you get no relief, a different type of treatment may be tried.

In the few cases where a very specific soft-tissue structure is affected, an anti-inflammatory injection may be offered. Injections that are effective may be repeated a couple of times.

Surgery is hardly ever needed, except in the rare cases when a specific tissue has been torn, broken or compressed so badly that it cannot heal and repair itself.

Stay active

Nearly everyone with arm pain due to soft-tissue problems is able to return to their usual activities in due course.

In general it is very important that you do not cease all activity. Rest and inactivity leads to muscle wasting and stiffness – too much rest is never useful for soft tissue problems. Movement stimulates blood flow and provides the chemicals needed for healing to take place. Movement also prevents muscle wasting. With soft tissue problems we need to remember the 'use-it-or-lose-it' phrase.

STAYING ACTIVE

"When the shoulder pain started, I thought I had better stop moving it. Then I discovered I was doing the opposite to what I should have been doing. As I gradually increased the movement, it started feeling better and the pain reduced."

Gradually increase your activity levels. Don't give up your usual activities, and also introduce some additional exercise, such as walking, swimming, cycling, running, yoga, tai chi – whatever you enjoy.

You have to allow some time for natural healing. The normal recovery course for soft tissue problems takes days or weeks. You can expect to have niggles and some setbacks as you improve. These can be frustrating, but you can do the very same things to help yourself as you did at the beginning. Continue to increase your activity levels. You may find you need to adjust what you do for a while. Don't let that lead you to rest up completely.

Action summary

Putting your plan into action:

- Take control –
  - Take responsibility for your recovery, making best use of help available
- Set realistic goals –
  - Give yourself a clear timeline for getting back to work and activity. Use weeks, not months
- Have a 'can-do' approach –
  - Avoid dwelling on what you can't do easily at present. You'll find you can do a lot of things – at work and leisure
- Talk with your health professional –
  - Discuss what you can do: sort out ways to get active and back to work. Give them permission to talk with your employer
- Increase activity –
  - Do a little more each day for a little longer. Schedule a gradual and steady increase in activity: do no more on good days and no less on bad days
- Changing your attitude and improving motivation
  - Don't get gloomy or anxious. Getting active will improve your confidence and you'll feel more positive
- Talk with your employer –
  - If your employer has not been in touch, make the first move. Temporary changes to your job are one of the best ways of making it possible to get

back to work: talk it through with your line manager

- Put it all together –
    - Make sure that you and your doctor and your employer all know what is happening and what you are planning. Tell them you want help to be a coper

Dealing with the 'ups and downs' of recovery

Remember that the process of getting better is usually an up and down one. Stay positive and don't give up

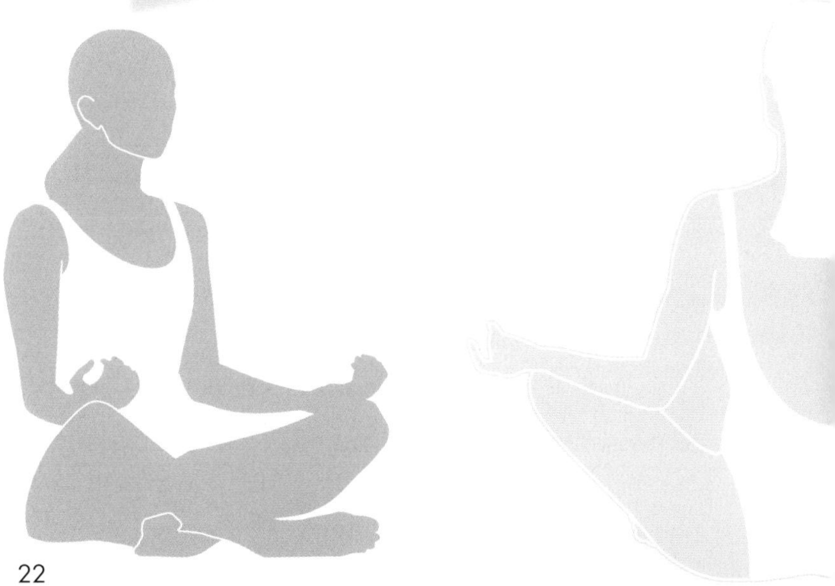

WHEN TO SEE YOUR DOCTOR

Although you can deal with a lot of arm problems yourself, there may be times when you are uncertain and feel the need to check. That's quite understandable. But you need to be realistic about what you expect from the doctor or therapist.

This is especially true in the early stages. It is very difficult to make an accurate diagnosis at the start, and most doctors will use what is known as a stepped care approach. Basically this means doing just what's needed and no more. Since most arm problems will settle with anti-inflammatory medication and exercise, that is what will be offered initially. It is only if things don't settle that further steps will be offered. This may involve physiotherapy or further medication. If the problem persists you may be sent for tests to establish the diagnosis, or you may be referred to a specialist. This will not apply to many people with arm pain.

Don't worry if you need to go through a few of these steps - it can take a little time. You should still try to carry on as normally as possible. Just check with your doctor or therapist whether there's anything you really should not be doing.

If you answer 'yes' to some of these questions, mention it to your doctor on your next visit:

Do you have a fever or chills? Do you have persistent tingling or numbness? Have you lost weight without any reason? Are you feeling really unwell? Is the part that hurts red, swollen, or hot? Do you have severe pain that is getting much worse?

Fit note

The fit note is a great idea, and can really help you. Why is this? Because it helps to focus on the things you can still do. Rather than the doctor having to sign you unfit for all work, you can be signed as fit for some work even if not your full job. Your doctor can help decide what parts of your job you can safely do. You need to take part in this by helping your doctor understand what you actually do at work.

The next bit is to sort out with your boss or line manager the tasks you can still do, and how best to adjust your job so you can keep working while you recover. This is much better than long periods off work and prevents things developing into a long-term problem. It makes sense to help yourself by asking for a fit note rather than expecting to be signed off sick.

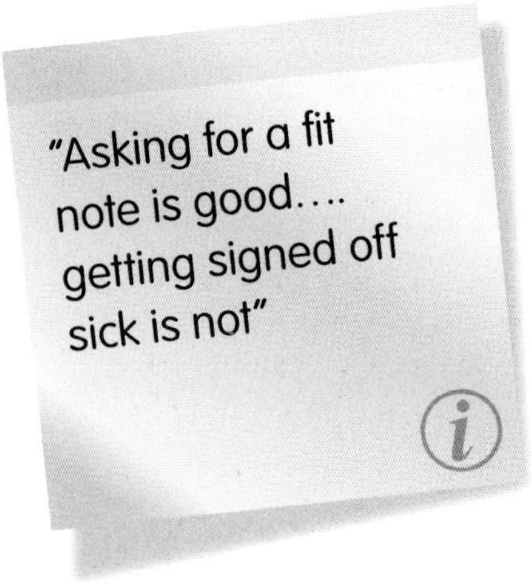

How to stay at work

Most people with arm problems can safely stay at work or get back to work with a bit of common sense and support at work. You may be told your arm pain is due to your work. This might be the case, but usually isn't. Even if it is, you should try to stay at work.

Obviously it depends on your work, but you may need to modify the way you do things to start with. It makes sense to avoid irritating the painful part of the arm too much – some discomfort is unavoidable and won't do any harm, but you'll want to pass up on really painful tasks.

There are various things you can do to help you stay at work. These are typical examples of what people say is helpful:

- change the tasks regularly
- avoid over-reaching
- take regular short breaks
- reduce weights
- get help from co-workers.

You can work out for yourself what is best for you, depending on what part of your arm is troubling you. Have a chat with your line manager and explain how you feel the job can be modified to help you out.

If that fails, you may need to look at the workplace itself, including tools and furniture. You may also discuss with your manager or safety rep whether a formal assessment is needed.

Two types:

One **avoids** activity, the other **copes**

- ☹ The 'avoider' becomes frightened, rests a lot, worries about the future and does too little
- The 'avoider' believes that hurting always means further damage – it doesn't
- ☺ The 'coper' accepts it will soon get better, stays positive, keeps active and stays at work
- The 'coper' knows the best thing is to get on with it

Who suffers most?

Avoiders: they have pain for longer, have more time off work and become disabled.

How do I become a **coper**?

- Don't get worried: it's not that serious...
- Control your pain: take the tablets!
- Stay active: this is better than over-resting
- Be patient: it's normal to get bad days
- Focus on work: get a little help from your friends

Mia's story shows how it should all be done. Simple as!